HUNGRY

OVERCOMING THE UNINTENDED HEALTH CONSEQUENCES OF THE PURSUIT OF OPTIMAL NUTRITION AND THE PERFECT BODY

BY JOEY LOTT

www.joeylott.com

Publishing services provided by 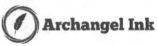 **Archangel Ink**

ISBN: 1518665942
ISBN-13: 978-1518665943

Table of Contents

4

The Cardinal Rule of Health

We live in a very strange time. While almost every other species on the planet understands and obeys the cardinal rule of health, an increasing number of humans have completely lost touch with it. As a result, we suffer. We suffer from symptoms including fatigue, digestive problems, insomnia, anxiety, bone loss, and inflammation. Sometimes these symptoms are severe to the point of being incapacitating. Sometimes they cause us to become bedridden. And many of these symptoms could be greatly diminished or completely eliminated if we would only follow the cardinal rule.

What is the cardinal rule of health? In a word: EAT.

A quick Google search on the keywords "benefits of eating less" turned up over 75 *million* results. Many of those results are specific to eating less of a particular type of food or nutrient, such as eating less sugar, less salt, or less meat. But millions upon millions of them would appear to be simply about eating less food. Period.

This should come as no surprise, of course. We are bombarded with messages about the "obesity epidemic" and how thin is sexy, healthy, and attractive. The message is almost always the same: eat less. We are told – either implicitly or explicitly -that eating less food or less of whole categories of food will help us to be healthier, happier, and more attractive. Heck, there are even claims that eating less food will make us *smarter*.

A trip to the grocery store can be very revealing. Products are marketed on the grounds that they contain less of everything. Less fat, fewer calories, less salt, no carbohydrates, no cholesterol, no sugar, and on and on. We are not only being told to eat less. We are *buying* it!

This would all be fine if it were actually true. If eating less actually made us healthier, smarter, more attractive, and happier, then it would be a wonderful service to us all that we are being convinced to do so. But in reality, eating less turns out to be far from the panacea that we are told. In fact, in more than a few cases, eating less makes us sicker and unhappy.

The reason? We are disobeying the cardinal rule of health.

If you have an opportunity, take some time to observe non-human animals. Watch the squirrels and chipmunks. Watch woodpeckers. Watch cows and horses. Watch hummingbirds. Watch chickens. What you'll undoubtedly notice is that they are often eating. I've cared for various livestock, and I've yet to encounter a pig or a chicken who turns down food when hungry. Heck, they don't even have to be hungry. They just eat. Same with cows. Same with goats. Same with horses.

But humans? Well, that's a whole other story. Humans routinely turn down food even when hungry. Humans will follow dubious advice such as drinking excessive water or eating large amounts of raw celery in order to curb hunger. Humans will avoid carbohydrates despite the fact that they have no energy and can't sleep through the night. Humans often have an unnecessarily complex relationship with food that seeks to sidestep the cardinal rule of health.

I know because I was one of those people. And like many people who don't eat enough, the sicker I felt, the more I restricted. I tried low-fat, low-carb, no grain, vegan, paleo, and on and on. Despite the promises of the diets, I kept feeling worse. Like many people, I assumed that I just hadn't found the perfect diet yet.

I was so sick that eating just about anything, even in very small amounts, made me feel uncomfortably bloated. I had terrible insomnia. I was suicidally depressed. I was cold all the time. I could barely walk. And this was despite my sincere and earnest efforts to improve my health by following the dietary advice of every proclaimed expert I could find. I tried really hard to find the right diet. But what none of the experts told me was the cardinal rule of health. *No one told me to just eat.*

What I didn't understand was that the reason the cardinal rule exists is because, first and foremost, getting enough calories is essential to health. And at the end of the day, if you don't eat enough calories, then it will make little difference whether those calories came from the "right" foods or the "wrong" foods. What matters is that you didn't get enough calories and you won't have enough energy to fuel the processes of your body. Plain and simple.

I began to eat more. Since I was unable to digest most foods at that time, I had to get really creative. I had to let go of all the restrictions. I had to focus on calories – the more the better. In this context, pure sugar is health food, which flies in the face of all the dietary dogma. But it turns out that obscene amounts of sugar played a major role in restoring vitality to my body. And as vitality returned, I became more capable of digesting more foods, which gave rise to even more vitality.

My own recovery was nothing short of miraculous, in my own view. Subsequently, I began to speak with people about my experiences in this regard. Through word of mouth, I began to speak with more people who have been sick with mysterious illnesses that doctors and other proclaimed experts didn't successfully treat. Over the past several years, I've spoken with about a hundred people who just can't seem to get well. In most cases, their health is deteriorating over time.

My purely unscientific observation in this matter has turned up a rather shocking statistic. Out of those hundred people, about 99 of them admit to under-eating and/or restricting whole categories of food. Out of the hundred people, about half have thus far refused to eat more and let go of restrictions, and their symptoms have generally not improved. The other half have agreed to eat more and let go of restrictions, and every one of those who began to eat more have seen some improvement, sometimes dramatic improvement.

As I have said, my survey is completely unscientific, but the results are so stark that it is impossible to disregard them. What the results seem to suggest quite strongly is that under-eating or food restriction, in any sense, may often be the cause of symptoms of sickness. And eating enough can often reverse these symptoms.

Starvation

I've just used the "S" word. Starvation. It's a strong word. And it ought to be, because it points to a very serious matter. But, unfortunately, we don't use the word very often any more in cases where it would be appropriate. Instead, we use words like "diet," "health food," "healthy," "fit," "pure," "anti-inflammatory," "high fiber," "sugar free," "fat free," and "low carb."

The confusion comes from the simple fact that many humans have deluded themselves into believing that the dietary requirements of a healthy human are *far* less than the demonstrable requirements. There are now incredible numbers of mainstream sources proposing to women and men that it is safe and sensible to eat as little as 1,200 calories a day for long periods of time in order to lose weight "safely." For example, the U.S. National Institutes of Health recommends a "healthy eating plan" suggesting that women can safely eat 1,000-1,200 calories a day, and men can safely eat 1,200-1,600 calories a day, in order to lose weight. And according to the U.S. government dietary recommendations, women may be able to maintain their weight and be healthy at a daily intake of just 1,600 calories, while men may be able to achieve the same with as little as 2,000 calories a day.

But these numbers and recommendations fly in the face of some of the only practical studies that have been done that monitor what the *actual* effects of calorie restriction are and what the *actual* caloric needs of adult humans are. The pre-eminent study is the Minnesota Starvation Experiment, which was conducted in 1944-1945.

The Minnesota Starvation Experiment included 36 young men who were initially healthy. They were recruited to study the effects of a prolonged state of semi-starvation. To begin with, the men were placed on a standardized maintenance diet of approximately 3,200 calories a day for 12 weeks. At the conclusion of this period, the men were determined to weigh in at just under their estimated "ideal" weights.

What followed was 24 weeks of semi-starvation, the goal of which was to reduce the men's weights by 25 percent. In order to achieve this goal, the men were started at 1,600 calories a day.

The outcomes were severe. At the conclusion of the 24 weeks, the men were emaciated, as was predicted. But the outcomes of the experiment were much more interesting than mere weight loss. To begin with, let's look at some of the physiological changes reported by the researchers. The basal (resting) metabolic rates of the participants were estimated to have fallen by as much as 40 percent. Their temperatures plummeted and their heart rates declined. Not surprisingly, they became intolerant of cold, fatigued, and easily exhausted – endurance reduced by *half.* They lost significant strength and their reflexes slowed. Some experienced anemia and edema (swelling).

The men's hair was falling out and their skin grew dry. They suffered from insomnia, tinnitus (ringing in the ears), and paresthesia (tingling and numbness). They lost sexual desire. The participants self-reported feelings of lack of concentration and decline in cognitive abilities. The study showed marked increases in hypochondria, meaning that the participants *felt sick* even though the researchers were not able to find the causes for those feelings.

Perhaps even more disturbing than the physiological symptoms were the emotional and psychological effects on the participants. The men were found to experience depression and anxiety. They became obsessive about food. They formed bizarre eating rituals. Despite the fact that they were severely underweight, many felt that they were overweight and developed distorted images of their own bodies (now known as body dysmorphism).

Following the starvation phase of the experiment, the participants underwent a restricted rehabilitation phase. During this phase, the men were divided into groups receiving 400, 800, 1,200, and 1,600 additional daily calories, respectively. Within the groups, the researchers made further subdivisions in order to monitor the effects not only of calories but also various nutrient ratios on re-feeding. The outcome of this phase was that over 12 weeks, those who were fed the most rehabilitated the most while those who were fed the least rehabilitated the least. The number of calories the men ate in a day was the single biggest factor determining the rate of recovery.

What is notable is that none of the men, not even those who were once again eating 3,200 calories a day – what had been enough previously to maintain a healthy weight – were able to recover fully in the 12 weeks.

Following the restricted rehabilitation phase, the men were placed on an eight-week unrestricted rehabilitation phase, during which they were given completely unrestricted access to as much food as they wanted. During this phase, the men routinely ate enormous amounts of food – some men eating as much as 11,000 calories a day for a time. And *still* at the end of the eight weeks, the men were only beginning to return to their pre-starvation weights and physical abilities.

What is also notable is that on average, once the men had fully recovered to their pre-starvation abilities, they had restored their original weight *plus* 10 percent. The majority of that additional weight was fat, not lean mass. This was seen to be a natural part of the recovery process. When the men continued to eat unrestrictedly, the majority of them returned to their pre-starvation weight and body composition nine months after re-feeding. This was accomplished without any restriction or additional exercise.

Based on studies such as the Minnesota Starvation Experiment, we have a list of symptoms that can be caused by starvation. Let's look at a short list of just some of those symptoms, in addition to the obvious likely outcome: weight loss.

- **Fatigue**
- **Reduction in endurance**
- **Weakness**
- **Insomnia**
- **Digestive problems**
- **Constipation**
- **Intolerance to cold (and sometimes heat)**
- **Anxiety and panic**
- **Irritability or moodiness**
- **Brain fog and lack of concentration**
- **Obsession (particularly about food)**
- **Body dysmorphia**
- **Immune deficiency**
- **Loss of sex drive**
- **Edema/swelling**
- **Shrinkage of organs, including heart, lungs, ovaries, and testes**
- **Hormonal imbalance**
- **Lowered basal metabolic rate**
- **Lowered temperature**

Now, before we put two and two together, let me share with you some words from Dr. Ancel Keys, director of the Minnesota Starvation Experiment. He wrote that "in an adult man, no appreciable rehabilitation can take place on a diet of 2,000 calories a day. The proper level is more like 4,000 kcal daily for some months." Considering that the men who participated in the study ate often considerably more than 4,000 calories a day during the unrestricted rehabilitation phase and *still* required many more months of unrestricted eating before returning to the pre-starvation state, Dr. Keys' words are a bit of an understatement. But he makes a clear point that the overwhelming majority of us have failed to understand for the past 70 years. He states the cardinal rule of *healing*, which is: eat. And eat *lots*.

Based on the evidence of the Minnesota Starvation Experiment and other subsequent investigations, it appears that younger people have higher caloric requirements than most adults over the age of 25. Men have higher caloric requirements than women who are neither pregnant nor lactating. And pregnant and lactating women have higher caloric requirements than men. Yet *most adults of either sex* have a daily caloric requirement of **at least 2,500 calories per day**.

There are exceptions, but you aren't likely to be one of them. The implication of this is that if you have been eating less than your minimum caloric requirements for any length of time, then you are likely experiencing a state of semi-starvation. If you are experiencing any of the symptoms attributable to starvation, then that reinforces the likelihood that you are experiencing semi-starvation. And here's the zinger: if you want to recover, then you likely need to eat *more* than your minimum caloric requirements for maintenance.

That's a lot to swallow. (Pardon the pun.) But these are the simple facts that almost no one is telling you. Still, there it is in black and white. The cardinal rule is very, very simple. Eat. Eat lots.

That's not what we're being told. We're being told to eat less – less calories, sugar, salt, fat, meat, carbohydrates, etc. And we're being told to rearrange the types of food we eat without giving particular concern to eating enough. But here are more words from Ancel Keys: "The character of the rehabilitation diet is important also, but unless calories are abundant, then extra proteins, vitamins and minerals are of little value."

My own experience validates Dr. Keys' statement. I was so sick that I couldn't stand for more than a minute at a time. I was reading book after book with dozens upon dozens of references to medical studies. The so-called experts were insisting that my problems were all because I was eating the wrong foods. They cited research they claimed proved that if only I would rearrange the types of foods that I ate to match their model (paleo, low carb, raw vegan, low fat, etc.), then I would feel better. But it wasn't until I finally ate enough consistently for long enough that I stopped getting sicker and started to actually feel better.

I'm not alone. I've seen the same thing time and time again. Those who refuse to eat enough keep trying to rearrange the proteins, fats, and carbohydrates in some sort of nightmarish game of musical chairs, and the overwhelming majority of them don't feel better. In fact, they keep getting sicker. But those who heed Dr. Keys' warning and focus on abundant calories first and foremost experience a reduction in symptoms – sometimes a complete remission.

Get Real

Some of us will already know that we are restricting calories, because we have been intentionally restricting for some reason or another. Yet others of us may be restricting calories inadvertently and not know. I was starving for years, even though I felt that I was gorging myself. Despite my attempts to eat as much as I could, I was barely clearing 1,600 calories on most days. Many people I communicate with are in the same boat. They don't realize how few calories they eat until they keep track.

If you do not know how many calories you eat on average, then I suggest that you begin to track your calories. (Those who are recovering from obsessive calorie tracking are often advised *not* to track calories. So please track calories only if doing so is not triggering for you. If tracking calories is triggering, then simply eat a *lot* of food.) There are several ways to do this. The easiest and most convenient way for most people is to use a food journal internet application such as cronometer.com, myfitnesspal.com, or fitday.com.

These applications generally make it easy to keep track not only of how many calories you eat, but also the macronutrient levels. I suggest you start tracking your calories for a few days to a week in order to see how much you are *actually* eating.

As we've already seen, actual calorie requirements are likely much higher than we've been led to believe. If you come up short, you'll know that you may benefit from experimenting with consistently eating more food.

According to the Minnesota Starvation Experiment, most men will require 3,200 calories per day for maintenance of health. Based on other studies, we may be able to lower that number to 3,000 for men over the age of 25. We can extrapolate from those results that most women will need at least 2,500 calories a day for maintenance. Pregnant and breastfeeding women and men under the age of 25 will need about 3,500 calories a day. And women under the age of 25 will need about 3,000 calories.

Note that those values are all for *maintenance of health*. But remember that Keys stated that by his estimates, men will require at least 4,000 calories per day for many months to recover after starvation or illness. So again, we can extrapolate that women over 25 will need 3,350 calories per day. Pregnant and breastfeeding women, as well as men under 25, will need 4,650 calories. And women under 25 will need 4,000 calories a day in order to recover.

So how do you measure up? Are you eating enough?

The Effects of Too Few Carbohydrates

We've already covered the problems of too few calories. And for most people most of the time, that is the number one problem they face. However, some people are committed to restricting entire macronutrients such that even if they increase the number of calories they eat, they will not recover properly. For that reason, in the following sections, we'll take a look at the effects of restricting specific macronutrients, starting with the restriction of carbohydrates.

Low-carb diets are all the rage these days. The Atkins diet is still alive and kicking, and updated low-carbohydrate diets are extremely popular, including variations on the Paleo diet as well as Mark Sisson's insanely popular Primal Blueprint diet. Advocates of low-carbohydrate diets suggest that the diets are powerful tools for weight loss, improving type 2 diabetes, and reversing metabolic syndrome. And very low-carbohydrate diets – known as ketogenic diets – have been used therapeutically to treat epilepsy.

Mark Sisson goes so far as to claim that eating 150 grams of carbohydrates or more a day will lead to "insidious weight gain." He and others claim that the ketones produced by the body during times of extreme carbohydrate restriction are the body's *preferred fuel source* (despite the evidence to the contrary). As a result, many actually advocate for eating less than 50 grams of carbohydrates a day in order to induce a state of ketosis.

For a very few people, low-carbohydrate diets are sustainable for the medium term. Some are even able to maintain a ketogenic diet for the medium term. But for the overwhelming majority of us, low-carbohydrate diets don't work. One of the biggest problems with a low-carbohydrate diet is that it can make obtaining enough calories extremely difficult. Although fat, which is often the primary source of calories on a low-carbohydrate diet, is a highly-concentrated energy source – more than twice as concentrated as carbohydrates – the simple fact is that fat and protein simply isn't palatable enough without sufficient carbohydrates for most people to eat sufficient calories.

While it is true that there may be a so-called "honeymoon phase" with a low-carbohydrate diet, for most people that phase wears off after a few weeks or months, or as long as a year or two in some rare cases. At that point, people crash with symptoms that include many of those seen in starvation, including digestive problems, insomnia, hair loss, irritability, brain fog, and so on.

Many low-carbohydrate advocates will claim that the problems that people experience on the diet are due to "not doing it right." This may be true, but by their own admission, "doing it right" is hard work. For example, in *The Art and Science of Low Carbohydrate Living*, experts Phinney and Volek describe some of the pitfalls that low-carb dieters fall into. One major pitfall that they identify is eating too much protein, which the body will then convert into glucose, preventing ketogenesis (which really ought to be a good indicator that ketogenesis is not the preferred state for the body). The implication here is that for a guy like me (at around 180 pounds) to eat a ketogenic diet, avoid eating too much protein, and get enough calories to avoid starvation, I would have to eat 280+ grams of fat per day. To put that in perspective, that's three sticks of butter *every day*. Don't get me wrong. I like butter, and I eat a lot. But three sticks every day? That's a bit much. Especially, if there are no potatoes to put it on.

Perhaps the main problem is that there really isn't any convincing evidence that carbohydrates are problematic for health, and there is plenty of evidence that carbohydrates can be very beneficial for health. So even if one was to successfully eat enough calories on a carbohydrate-restricted diet, it's not clear that there would be any benefits. And, in most cases, it doesn't turn out to be sustainable. Most people crash on low-carbohydrate diets sooner or later.

The bottom line with regard to carbohydrates is that if you really want to restrict them, then in *most* cases it is advisable to first eat an unrestricted diet with adequate calories for long enough to restore health. And for most people, that will mean consistently eating many thousands of calories a day (as in something approaching or exceeding Dr. Keys' recommended 4,000 calories a day) for many months or even years. At that point, if you truly want to experiment with a low-carbohydrate diet, then you will be in a better position to try it out.

The Effects of Too Little Protein

Most diets with enough calories are unlikely to contain too little protein, but it can and does happen under various circumstances. I was a long-time adherent to the vegan diet, which eschews all meat, dairy, eggs, and other animal foods. And the most common question that non-vegans would pose was, "How do you get your protein?" In reaction, like many vegans, I completely dismissed the real concerns that can arise in the face of too little dietary protein.

Protein is the most abundant macronutrient in the human body. It is essential to life, most popularly known as the basis of skeletal muscle. But protein does so much more than make bigger biceps. Protein is a major component of all the organs of the body, skin, hair, and even bone. Protein is needed for building and transporting hormones. It is needed for building the components of the immune system. Protein is an essential part of red blood cells. And even nucleic acid, which is the way in which our genetic information is encoded, requires protein.

Conventional recommendations suggest that adults need approximately 0.8 grams of protein per kilogram of body mass in order to avoid deficiency. What that means is that someone like me, weighing about 180 pounds (or 82 kilograms) needs around 65 grams of protein daily as a minimum. And increased physical activity will increase the demand for dietary protein. So if I'm lifting heavy things, for example, then my body will need more.

Although it is easy to dismiss the conventional recommendations as being too conservative, I find that they offer a good minimum target. Less than 0.8 grams per kilogram often starts to produce symptoms of protein deficiency.

The good news is that it is very difficult to dramatically undershoot minimum protein requirements when eating enough calories. Even if one were to rely on orange juice – which is relatively low in protein – for all of one's caloric requirements, it would still provide nearly enough protein. For example, in order for me to meet my caloric needs (which we will estimate at around 3,200 calories per day), that would require that I drink nearly two gallons of orange juice a day, providing approximately 64 grams of protein!

So for a person who is primarily sedentary and who is eating enough each day, it is very difficult to get too little protein. The biggest danger to most people is in eating too little, which means both a caloric deficit *and* a potential protein deficit. So eating enough calories should always be the main priority.

Even when eating enough calories, it is reasonable to give some attention to the quality of the protein that you eat, because even though in the rather extreme example I gave of eating nothing but orange juice, despite the fact that it would provide enough protein, the *quality* of the protein is not very good.

Proteins are composed of amino acids. Different types of protein have different ratios of amino acids. Our bodies are capable of synthesizing most types of amino acids, but there are eight that it cannot. These eight are called *essential* amino acids. Most plant foods (and I know that vegans everywhere cringe when I write this) are deficient in some essential amino acid or another. So it is *theoretically* possible to obtain all the amino acids from plant foods, but in reality, animal proteins are much higher quality. So the easiest way to ensure adequate *quality* protein is to eat an omnivorous diet that includes a variety of both plant and animal foods *in sufficient quantity.*

Although frank protein deficiency is considered to be rare among Western populations, there are some populations who are at risk for some degree of deficiency, including the elderly, athletes, injured people, vegans (especially raw vegans), and those who are sick or recovering from semi-starvation. In all these cases, the protein requirements are significantly increased. In other words, if you have been sick or if you've ever been in semi-starvation mode and you aren't feeling on top of the world just yet, then you may need to increase your protein intake to avoid a deficiency.

When we think of protein deficiency, images of starving African children probably pop into our minds. In the condition known as Kwashiorkor, which occurs when there are sufficient calories but insufficient protein, the sufferer may develop classic signs such as edema of the belly, fatty liver, and flaky skin. But even without the classic signs, it is possible to suffer from mild to moderate protein deficiency. Some symptoms include apathy, diarrhea, irritability, anorexia, thinning hair, tooth loss, and dermatitis.

Ironically, protein deficiency can create the conditions in which one has a diminished appetite. So if you are feeling unwell, you lack appetite, and your protein intake is less than, say 1 gram per kilogram of body mass, then you may benefit from a moderate increase in quality protein intake. If well-tolerated, then dairy and egg protein are generally very high quality.

The Effects of Too Little Fat

There is a tremendous amount of confusion in the public debate about dietary fat. Depending on which camps you fall into, you may believe that saturated fat is the cause of all health problems; you may believe that polyunsaturated fat is the cause of all health problems; or you may believe that *any* fat is bad for your health.

The problems with fat phobia of any sort are many. The greatest danger of fat phobia is that it may lead to insufficient caloric intake. In extreme cases, people restrict all dietary fat, which vastly reduces likelihood of eating enough. Fat is more than twice as energy-dense as either protein or carbohydrates. So for every gram of fat that you don't eat, you have to eat more than twice that much of carbohydrates or protein in order to compensate. For this reason alone, adding moderate amounts of dietary fat is a great help in recovery from sickness.

And, of course, dietary fat simply *tastes good*. Plain potatoes? No thank you. But fried in butter? Yum. So the addition of dietary fat tends to make foods more palatable, which also enables you to eat more calories.

Generally speaking, fats are categorized as saturated, monounsaturated, and polyunsaturated. And *all* natural fats contain some of each type, though the ratios will vary. Animal fats such as butter, lard, or tallow contain relatively higher amounts of saturated fat versus most (though not all) seed or nut oils. Most seed or nut oils are high in polyunsaturated fats with the exception of tropical oils. And olive oil contains large amounts of monounsaturated fat, which is also found in significant quantities in some animal fats.

While some groups like to demonize saturated fat and other groups like to demonize polyunsaturated fat, the truth is that both are necessary for health. A deficiency in either type can produce health problems. Saturated fats are necessary for a tremendous number of functions in the body, not the least of which is the creation of hormones. And a certain type of polyunsaturated fats called omega-3 fatty acids are necessary for a whole host of functions in the body, as well. So it is a terrible idea to attempt to *eliminate* either type of fat.

At present, the evidence seems to point to the likelihood that polyunsaturated omega-6 fatty acids, which happen to predominate in the majority of nut and seed oils (excepting tropical oils like coconut and palm), are inflammatory and may lead to health problems when consumed in *excess*. Therefore, it is sensible to include a variety of natural, healthy, palatable fats such as butter and olive oil in moderation in the diet. Natural fats that occur in real foods such as meats, dairy, and olives contain enough of saturated, monounsaturated, and polyunsaturated fats to maintain health.

Yet another reason that adequate dietary fat intake is important is because it is necessary for the absorption of fat-soluble vitamins such as vitamins A, D, E, and K. And, in fact, natural fats are often the best or only reliable sources of some of these essential vitamins.

Dietary fat deficiency can lead to a whole host of symptoms directly or indirectly, due to malabsorption issues. Some of the most common symptoms of fat deficiency include dry skin, feeling cold, cognitive difficulties, hormonal imbalance, achy joints, brittle nails, dry hair, constipation, digestive problems, irritability, depression, and weakness.

Of course, you needn't go out of your way to include essential fats in your diet. As long as you eat sufficient calories and include moderate amounts of naturally-occurring fats in your diet, you will meet your dietary fat requirements. So instead of opting for low- or non-fat products or forgoing the butter, eat full-fat foods, and include butter or other natural fat sources to taste in your foods.

The Effects of a Plant Based Diet

Plant-based diets, or vegan diets, are increasingly popular these days. Advocates promote the diets for health, environmental, and ethical reasons. I ate a vegan diet for a variety of reasons for 17 years, and so I am very familiar with the concerns that motivate such a choice. And yet, the simple fact is that despite what we may want to believe, the evidence is strongly suggestive that a vegan diet makes it much more challenging to recover or maintain good health, when compared to a vegetarian (which includes dairy and eggs) or an omnivorous diet. The full critique of the vegan diet is beyond the scope of this book, and I have written another book on the subject titled *Vegan Recovery* for those interested in exploring the subject in more detail. However, in this section, I'd like to explore some of the challenges that a plant-based diet present for health.

To begin with, vegan diets are inherently nutrient-deficient, as there are several key nutrients that occur *only* in animal foods. Of particular note are vitamins A and

B12. While the human body is theoretically capable of converting carotenoids such as beta-carotene to true vitamin A (retinol), in practice the conversion is generally poor. And in some people, the conversion is extremely poor or non-existent. Thus, the only truly reliable sources of vitamin A are animal foods such as butter, eggs, and liver.

Symptoms of vitamin A deficiency include vision problems (such as poor night vision), dry eyes, inflammation of the eyes, immune deficiency with particular susceptibility to urinary or respiratory infections, and skin dryness or roughness.

Vitamin B12 is perhaps the most common deficiency in vegans since there are no reliable plant-based sources of B12, whereas nearly all animal foods contain the vitamin. Deficiencies in this vitamin can lead to symptoms including weakness, fatigue, sore tongue, easy bruising or bleeding, diarrhea, constipation, digestive problems, anemia, jaundice, cognitive difficulties, anxiety, lightheadedness, and paranoia.

Iron deficiency is not as common as A or B12 deficiency, but it can happen on a vegan diet since plant sources of iron (non-heme) are poorly absorbed by the body. Animal foods contain more heme iron than plant foods, making them better sources that are more easily absorbed. Symptoms of iron deficiency can include brittle nails, sore tongue, cracks in the side of the mouth, immune deficiency, fatigue, cognitive difficulties, shortness of breath, and pale skin.

Vegan diets also create a complete absence of dietary cholesterol. Despite the demonization of the substance, cholesterol is important for health. Cholesterol is essential for cell structure, bile production, hormone creation, and the insulation of nerves. In fact, if there is insufficient dietary cholesterol, then the body will manufacture cholesterol from sugars. So eating too little cholesterol places additional demands on the body, and may even lead to what some are now referring to as cholesterol deficiency symptoms, including depression, anxiety, impulsivity, cognitive difficulties, irritability, digestive problems, and even aggression.

Although vegan advocates generally hate to admit it, the simple fact is that plant proteins are not as high quality as animal proteins. Although a vegan diet can theoretically provide for the protein needs of a healthy person, they make it more challenging to provide for the increased protein needs of people who are recovering from illness or otherwise simply not feeling 100 percent.

Finally, vegan diets are more likely than omnivorous diets to contain high ratios of inflammatory polyunsaturated omega-6 fatty acids to other fats in the diet. That can lead to health problems. This is not an inherent problem with the vegan diet, since it is possible to eat plant-based fats that contain favorable amounts of saturated, monounsaturated, and omega-3 fatty acids, but the most common fats in vegan diets, including seed oils (corn, soy, canola, sunflower, safflower, and so on) and most nuts and seeds, are high in polyunsaturated omega-6 fatty acids, while low in other types of healthy fats.

Although it does seem true that some people are able to experience good health in the short to medium term on a *well-planned* vegan diet, most people seem to have a better chance at recovery when eating an omnivorous diet that includes adequate calories, fats, fat-soluble vitamins, cholesterol, quality protein, vitamin B12, and iron among other important vitamins and minerals that are generally easier to acquire from animal foods.

Digestive Problems

Perhaps one of the most common symptoms of under-eating or restriction that I encounter fall under the catch-all of digestive problems. This can include bloating, excessive mucus, indigestion, cramping, sluggish digestion, diarrhea, constipation, and intolerance of various types of foods that develop over time (versus genetic predispositions). I know these symptoms intimately because I lived with them for more than a decade.

Digestive problems often lead to a vicious cycle of further restrictions. Yet the more one restricts, the worse the symptoms become! In the hopes of repairing our digestive issues, many of us turn to specialized diets such as Gut and Psychology Syndrome (GAPS) diet, Selective Carbohydrate Diet, autoimmune Paleo, zero carb, raw vegan, and so on. While there are occasionally people who experience miraculous healings using these specialized diets, the vast majority end up getting sicker over time. Eventually, most people make the rounds through all the different types of special diets, combining various elements of them until they are reduced to eating little more than a handful of "safe" foods. And most keep getting sicker.

Nearly everyone I speak with reports the same pattern of worsening digestive symptoms over time as they restrict more and more foods. The more foods they eliminate, the more foods they react to. In my own experience, I eventually felt so bloated and uncomfortable after eating *anything* – even after drinking sips of water – that I gave up on eating and drinking water for a week! I was thoroughly exhausted from trying so much to find something that I could eat.

Hopefully by now, you can already see how restricting (whether intentional or not) calories and/or macronutrients can lead to this vicious cycle. Reductions in calories can lead to digestive problems as metabolic rate slows, digestive transit slows, temperature drops, and energy levels plummet. Deficiencies in any macronutrient can lead to problems, as well. For example, protein deficiency will lower appetite. Deficiencies in fat can cause digestive weakness and constipation. And carbohydrate deficiencies can also cause problems ranging from nausea to lowered appetite to constipation or diarrhea.

Unfortunately, most of the time we misinterpret these symptoms as evidence that we should further restrict. But the more that we restrict (intentionally or unintentionally), the worse the symptoms become. As our symptoms worsen, we will likely read more books and articles on the Internet that advocate for special diets that cause us to restrict even more. Soon enough, we'll have cut out all grain, all starch, all sugar, fat, and so forth. Cutting out or drastically restricting *any* foods reduces the ease with which you can eat enough calories.

Of course, some people simply have little choice but to restrict some foods because they are genuinely intolerant of them. For example, people with symptomatic Celiac disease will generally be better off eliminating gluten-containing foods, which means that people with Celiac disease will need to be creative in order to eat enough food. But people who do not have Celiac disease will not gain any benefit by eliminating gluten-containing foods. Even people who have the genetic predisposition for Celiac disease will not necessarily gain any benefits from eliminating gluten if they are not symptomatic, since one may have the genetic markers for Celiac without actually have the active form of the disease. The same goes for *any* restriction of foods. It is only wise to restrict if there is a genuine need and benefit in doing so. Otherwise, the restriction is likely to contribute to decreases in calories and possibly deficiencies in macronutrients.

In my own unscientific observations, I have noticed that when people take the advice to eat enough on a consistent basis, digestive problems almost always improve or disappear entirely. That does not mean that in every case the problems will disappear overnight or that the reintroduction of foods may not sometimes cause temporary unpleasant symptoms, but it does mean that with consistent, creative efforts to find ways to eat enough that work for the individual, symptoms such as bloating, cramping, constipation, diarrhea, sluggishness, and general digestive weakness tend to improve over time, usually with significant improvements happening within weeks.

Edema

Edema, or water retention, is a very common effect of insufficient caloric intake and/or insufficient protein intake. Dieters often refer to this as dieter's edema or the "whoosh effect," in which water retention can sometimes be so extreme that one can leave temporary indentations in the skin by pressing lightly with a finger.

I communicated with a woman named Angela who was experiencing, among other symptoms, edema so severe that she ended up in the emergency room on several occasions. The emergency room employees remarked at what a dramatic accumulation of fluid she was exhibiting. Her abdomen and her legs would literally swell to about twice their normal size. This happened so often that when she was not swelling, her skin began to sag.

Angela was eating a dramatically restricted diet because her many healthcare providers were suggesting that she limit and even completely eliminate many foods that tests had shown she was allergic to. As a result, her daily caloric intake was below 1,500 calories, sometimes even below 1,000 calories. She had trouble sleeping, she felt anxious, she experienced panic attacks, and her energy levels had fallen dramatically.

None of Angela's many healthcare providers had suggested to her that caloric restriction (and insufficient macronutrient intake) could cause any of her symptoms. Instead, they kept suggesting that she further restrict her diet as she developed more food intolerances.

I worked with Angela to help reduce her stress and anxiety levels through some simple meditative techniques, which offered some relief, but I felt strongly that in order to really recover, she would need to eat much more food. I encouraged her to eat more over the course of many months of communicating. She was reluctant at first, but eventually she began to increase her caloric intake and include more foods that she had previously been restricting.

As she began to eat more and continued to practice the simple techniques for relaxation that I had given her, she ceased to swell up. Her skin regained its elasticity and returned to normal appearance. She began to sleep through the night. She ceased to experience panic attacks, and her anxiety levels dramatically decreased.

Although Angela's edema was the most dramatic I have seen, this symptom is common among those I communicate with. I experienced uncomfortable water retention myself when I was at my worst health and eating next to nothing. During that time, I felt that I couldn't drink any water because my body was holding on to every drop of it. I could swing my abdomen from side to side and hear a swishing sound.

In every single case so far in my experience, edema improves by eating enough food. Sometimes there is a stage during re-feeding in which edema begins to occur. When this occurs, it goes the quickest when one continues to eat and rest as much as possible. Further restriction exacerbates the problem.

Anxiety

Anxiety is an *extremely* common symptom of insufficient nutrition (calories or macronutrients). Almost every single person I communicate with who is under-eating or restricting macronutrients experiences some form of anxiety, which can range from mild feelings to tension and discomfort to full-blown de-realization and panic. Strangely, no one else has ever suggested to most of us that eating more food could help. In fact, many healthcare professionals, as well as friends and family, suggest the opposite – that further restriction may help. But the more that people restrict, the worse the symptoms of anxiety become.

What we call anxiety is actually a physiological phenomenon. It is the result of various physical changes in the body, including the increased production of stress hormones such as adrenalin and cortisol. And what very few people seem to realize is that insufficient calories or insufficient macronutrients can lead to these stressful changes.

Eating too few calories provides too little energy for the body. The result is that the body has to break down protein and fat in the body in order to sustain itself. And eventually, the body will have to lower the metabolic rate in order to run off of less energy. The result is that the body is running inefficiently, relying on backup survival systems of energy production that create inflammation and excess stress hormones in the body.

Deficiencies of any of the macronutrients can also produce stress. Too little fat can release stored up polyunsaturated free fatty acids, which oxidize easily, meaning increases in inflammation. Too little fat can also eventually deplete sex hormones as well as nerve sheath (called myelin), leading to feelings of anxiety.

Carbohydrate restriction also causes the body to adapt by relying on backup systems of energy production. These backup systems use stress hormones, which can produce feelings of anxiety in the body. Carbohydrate restriction may also deplete hormones in the body.

Protein deficiency is well-known to produce a wide range of mood disturbances, including not only depression and apathy, but also anxiety. Adequate quality protein is necessary to build and maintain a healthy nervous system, and when protein intake is too low, the body cannot repair and maintain the nervous system properly.

Like many people who under-eat, I used to experience extreme anxiety and even paranoia. I had no idea that the way I felt was connected to eating too little. I tried many dietary changes, including those that claim to solve anxiety such as GAPS or various Ayurvedic lifestyle changes, but nothing helped. I eventually learned how to know peace and not become shaken up by the feelings, but it wasn't until I began to eat enough consistently that the feelings of anxiety themselves began to diminish significantly.

Lyme Disease

I lived with chronic Lyme disease for a number of years, and during that time, I experienced a worsening of every symptom I had ever had, including insomnia, digestive disturbances, lack of appetite, irritability, and on and on. I tried every natural approach to healing that I could find, including herbs, diets, saunas, and so forth, but it wasn't until I began to eat enough food that I finally began to heal.

After recovering my health, I wanted to give back by offering help to others who suffer with the condition. Many of the people with whom I communicate have been diagnosed with chronic Lyme disease, testing positive for infections with Lyme bacteria as well as multiple co-infections. And thus far, *every single one* eats far too little. Oftentimes, people are eating restricted diets because they have either been prescribed a restrictive diet by a Lyme literate doctor, or because they have decided to restrict their diets based on recommendations they have read.

The diets that people with chronic Lyme disease attempt range from so-called anti-inflammatory diets to Gerson therapy diets to GAPS to Paleo to raw vegan and so on. But what they always have in common (at least thus far in my experience) is insufficient calories. I communicated with a man recently who was eating 1,500 calories a day. I communicated with a woman recently who was eating 1,200 calories a day. Both were already underweight. Both were fatigued, anxious, weak, and irritable. Nobody told them that eating too few calories could produce their symptoms.

I have read a *lot* of books about Lyme disease treatments, and the majority of them recommend restricted diets. The *only* book on the subject that I know of that stresses the importance of eating *enough* calories is my book, *Healing Chronic Lyme Disease Naturally*. So it is no wonder that the majority of people who have been diagnosed with chronic Lyme disease are eating too little. And because they are eating too little, it is little wonder why they are not feeling better.

Eating too little can lead to nearly every single symptom of chronic Lyme disease. Of course, eating enough will not always resolve every symptom, but without eating enough, it is completely unreasonable to expect that symptoms will improve. Whatever other treatments one may choose in order to treat chronic Lyme disease, eating enough is absolutely essential.

Muscle Control

I communicated with a woman named Mona who had developed extreme sensitivities to some chemical products, beginning with a type of glue that she had used in her occupation. Over the course of a year, the sensitivities grew worse until she was unable to step foot in a room of her house where a few of the products that had been made with the glue were stored. If she entered the room, she began feeling dizzy and weak. Overall, her health declined. She grew lethargic and irritable. Perhaps most notable was that she began to lose control over her muscles, the most significant of which was she couldn't control when she urinated. This was, understandably, a very upsetting experience for her.

Through conversation, I discovered that Mona had a lifetime history of dieting and food restriction – not uncommon among women (and men). She was underweight at the time, and her caloric intake was insufficient even for maintaining her health, much less healing. Not only was she obviously calorie deficient, but she was also clearly not eating enough protein.

I recommended some simple dietary adjustments. Primarily, I suggested that she eat a lot more food, emphasizing calorie-dense, palatable foods such as ice cream, cookies and cake, whenever she desired. I suggested that she add butter to foods. And I suggested that she increase her protein intake by eating more dairy, eggs, and meat.

I also gave Mona some simple relaxation exercises to do that specifically are designed to help desensitize the over-reactive limbic system, which I suspected was playing a role in the dramatic experiences she had specific to the room with the products.

After only a month, she was able to spend time in the room that had previously troubled her without reaction. And her muscle control returned. She no longer experienced any incontinence, despite the fact that doctors had told her that they could do nothing to help her.

Mona is not an anomaly. Many people I speak with develop tremors, uncoordinated movements, shakiness, poor reflex response, and loss of specific motor function. And when people begin to eat enough consistently, these symptoms typically improve.

Osteoporosis

I have spoken with a number of people who have been diagnosed with osteoporosis, which refers to a severe loss of bone density. Their doctors, endocronologists, and other healthcare providers often sought to give them estrogen drugs to increase bone density, but several of the people had instances of breast cancer in their families that gave them reason to be concerned about taking the drugs. When they sought out alternative treatments, they usually came up with the same sorts of advice: supplement with calcium, magnesium, vitamin D, vitamin K, vitamin A, and boron; take fish oil supplements; do more weight-bearing exercise. And while all the nutritional and lifestyle advice may (or may not) be reasonable, it overlooks a major contributing factor to osteoporosis. What is that factor? You guessed it – eating too little.

The fact of the matter is that the connection between calorie restriction, macronutrient deficiencies, and loss of bone density is now a well-known phenomenon among researchers. In both laboratory and human studies, the evidence is strong that calorie restriction correlates to instances of osteoporosis. For example, a study at the Washington University School of Medicine found that subjects who restricted calories lost an average of 2.2 percent of spinal and hip bone density, whereas an exercise-only group and a control group lost no bone density.

Unfortunately, as of this writing, I cannot report on any anecdotal evidence of those whom I have communicated with recovering from osteoporosis by eating enough. But the reason is simply that, to date, those who I have communicated with on the subject have refused to eat enough. More often than not, the reasons cited for why they won't eat more is that they are concerned about gaining weight.

However, the evidence is quite strong that the single best treatment for osteoporosis (or osteopenia) in cases of calorie restriction is re-feeding with adequate calories (and adequate levels of all macronutrients). It is well-known among those who study eating disorders, such as anorexia nervosa that involve calorie restriction, that the best treatment for any resulting bone density loss is re-feeding. Despite this fact, healthcare practitioners rarely seem to investigate caloric restriction as a likely cause in many cases of bone density loss, and as a result, they rarely recommend eating more as a treatment.

Don't Fear Food

In the preceding sections, I've explored just a handful of the common complications and health challenges that I encounter with people who are eating too little. What is shocking is that due to a gross misunderstanding of the actual caloric and nutritional needs of the human body, far too many healthcare providers are failing to address what is likely to be the underlying cause of many of the symptoms – under-eating or macronutrient restriction. In fact, with the current trends in dietary advice, many sick people are being advised to further restrict their diets. The result is predictable: declining health.

But Ancel Keys said it clearly when he stated: "The character of the rehabilitation diet is important, also, but unless calories are abundant, then extra proteins, vitamins and minerals are of little value." If you eat too little, then regardless of the nutrient density of the food or the ratios of nutrients, the diet will fail to support true recovery. And any caloric deficiency is likely to contribute to declining health.

Put simply, a great many illnesses and mysterious symptoms that people today are experiencing are likely the result of starvation. Yet, because we are being advised to eat less of everything, the problems worsen over time.

If you presently eat too few calories, or if you have *ever* restricted and not fully restored weight and metabolic health through adequate rest and re-feeding, then it is reasonable to assume that any symptoms that you experience *may* be due to inadequate nutrition. Therefore, the most reasonable treatment for most symptoms is to eat more and get adequate rest.

Of course, this advice flies in the face of conventional advice, but 70 years ago, the Minnesota Starvation Experiment demonstrated clearly that insufficient caloric intake leads to a wide range of symptoms, including both physiological and psychological symptoms. Furthermore, full recovery requires eating large numbers of calories for long periods of time. Therefore, *any* continued restriction of calories of macronutrients will prevent a full recovery.

Unfortunately, the majority of us are now afraid of many foods, and this is a major obstacle to recovery. Between the American Heart Association, the American Cancer Society, the federal dietary recommendations, Dr. McDougall, Dr. Ornish, Paleo advocates, vegan advocates, Gary Taubes, and millions of other dietary pundits, we are afraid of just about everything. Millions of people are now counting calories, reducing fat, ditching carbohydrates, eliminating sugar, going grain-free, and replacing meals with green smoothies – all in an attempt to improve health. But what many of us are inadvertently doing is starving ourselves.

Some who starve themselves look the part – emaciated, skin on bones, sunken eyes, and so forth. But there are a great many people who are starving themselves, yet still appear to themselves and to others as "overweight." The problem is that starvation doesn't have only one appearance. Severe starvation will invariably lead to dramatic loss of muscle and fat mass, but all the metabolic and physiological effects of starvation can be present even if a person appears to have large amounts of adipose tissue.

Many attempt to lose weight through the "eat less, exercise more" paradigm. Others attempt to lose weight by adhering to extreme dietary practices, such as ketogenic diets. While these approaches may work in the short term, the long-term effects are now well-known. What happens is that over time, it becomes harder and harder to lose weight even when resorting to extreme measures.

Why might that be? Well, if we once again look to the Minnesota Starvation Experiment, then we have a pretty strong clue. The researchers attempted to induce 2.5 pounds of weight loss in each man for every week during the semi-starvation phase. According to the standard calories in = calories out model that is still popular today, a reduction of 3,500 calories below maintenance levels will create a loss of one pound of mass. In other words, to achieve 2.5 pounds of loss per week, all that should have been necessary would have been a 1,250 calorie reduction per day per man. The maintenance levels as established in the first phase of the experiment determined that the men required an average of 3,200 calories per day to maintain their weight. That means that if each man ate 1,950 calories per day during the semi-starvation phase, he should have been expected to lose 2.5 pounds per week for every week.

But the experiment showed that the calories in = calories out model didn't work. The researchers adjusted the daily calories of the men in order to reach their target weight loss, and they had to average 1,600 calories in order to get the men to lose enough weight. And, not only that, but in the end, the average weight loss was 37 pounds instead of 60 pounds, as should have been expected. What the researchers found was that the longer the men starved, the less weight they lost. And eventually, in the last weeks of the semi-starvation phase, no man lost weight. In fact, several men *gained* weight despite being placed on extremely restricted diets.

What the experiment found was that basal metabolic rate dropped by an average of 40 percent. That meant that the men were expending far less energy. Their bodies were adjusting to keep them alive under extreme circumstances.

Ironically, the more one attempts to starve oneself, the lower the metabolic rate drops. Then, even once food is reintroduced (*if* it is reintroduced in adequate quantities), the body will gain weight – especially fat – at a quick rate. It may take many months or even years of consistent adequate caloric intake before the body readjusts to non-starvation conditions, and resets the metabolic rate and the body composition.

The *only* diet known to achieve recovery is an *unrestricted* diet with adequate calories and all macronutrients. Remember that during the unrestricted rehabilitation phase of the Minnesota Starvation Experiment, the men were sometimes eating more than 11,000 calories a day. It was common for the men to eat large meals and still feel unsatisfied. They would sometimes eat again only half an hour after finishing a large meal. All of these behaviors are popularly judged as "unhealthy." However, in the context of recovery from starvation, these behaviors are absolutely essential.

Fearing food makes it nearly impossible to recover from starvation and sickness. The reason is that the body may require inordinate amounts of calories and nutrients, and if one greatly restricts the types of foods that one will eat, it is extremely difficult to eat enough. As an example, let's consider that the body of someone who is recovering may occasionally require 10,000 calories in a day. If that person excludes sugar, refined foods, and gluten (all commonly-restricted foods), then you can imagine how difficult it might be to eat 10,000 calories. To put this in perspective, consider that a meal with a large 12 ounce steak, three baked potatoes with generous amounts of butter and sour cream, and some helpings of "healthy" non-starchy vegetables with butter contains only about 2,000 calories. Go ahead and try to eat that five times in a day. You'd have a heck of a time.

But, if instead you eat an unrestricted diet that not only includes steaks, potatoes, butter, and cream, but also ice cream, milk shakes, brownies, bread, apple cobbler, maple syrup, and the like, then you'll suddenly have a much easier time eating enough.

As someone who was formerly terrified of sugar, starch, refined foods, meat, fat, grain, dairy, and just about every other sort of food, I know how difficult this advice can be to swallow (sorry for the pun). But as someone who tried every other dietary suggestion under the sun and kept getting sicker, and as someone who finally recovered after eating unrestrictedly of all the "bad" foods, I am convinced that none of the "bad" foods are actually all that bad. In fact, in the context of re-feeding for recovery, many of the "bad" foods are some of the very best because they allow for a massive intake of calories that simply wouldn't be possible with so-called "good" foods alone.

I have seen the same thing happen over and over again. People are afraid of foods, with long lists of bad foods and short lists of good foods. Meanwhile, they get sicker and sicker, continuing to move more foods from the good column to the bad column. And the only thing that finally helps them to recover is to eat liberally of all the foods – good or bad.

In practice, some foods tend to be tremendously valuable in re-feeding. Not surprisingly, the foods that tend to be the most helpful are those that by conventional thinking are "bad." Some of the most powerful foods for recovery are sugar (including all types of sugar such as cane sugar or maple syrup), starch, saturated fat such as found in butter or coconut oil, salt (liberal use of salt can often dramatically improve digestion), red meat, eggs, gelatin, refined grain flour, and cream. Put these things together and you end up with chocolate chip cookies, ice cream, and home-fried potatoes.

The biggest mistake that people make apart from intentional calorie restriction is to restrict "bad" foods on an ideological basis. Many people have been so inculcated by the dietary pundits that they are terrified of refined flours, insisting on eating only sprouted whole grains. Or they won't eat granulated sugar, compromising by eating only whole fruits instead. The reason this is a mistake is that in the context of re-feeding for recovery, the most important qualities in a food are caloric density and palatability. Unfortunately, whole grains and whole fruits don't fare so well on those accounts, whereas refined flours and granulated sugar are perfect examples of ideal recovery foods. Put them together with some eggs, a stick of butter, and some cocoa powder, and you've got brownies, which may be king among recovery foods (or possibly a close second to ice cream, depending on your sensibilities and preferences).

In practice, are there any foods that genuinely ought to be on the "bad" list? It would seem that the answer to this is, "it depends." The number one priority should always be eating enough calories and a balance of macronutrients. If you eat at least 3,000-4,000 calories a day during re-feeding, and you eat a variety of real foods, then that is what is most important. However, once that matter is taken care of, it is sensible to keep a few foods in moderation.

The aim of re-feeding is three-fold. First and foremost, you want to supply enough calories. Secondly, you want to supply enough nutrients (macro and micro). And thirdly, you want to nourish your metabolism. The third goal is where some "bad" foods may come into play. There are some foods that may suppress metabolic health. The primary culprit seems to be polyunsaturated fat. Of course, as we've already seen, it is undesirable (not to mention completely impractical) to entirely eliminate all polyunsaturated fat from one's diet. And in small amounts, polyunsaturated fat appears to be important for health. But excessive polyunsaturated fat may be problematic. The most common sources of polyunsaturated fats in most diets these days come from seed oils such as soy, corn, canola, safflower, and sunflower oil. So for the purposes of recovery, it is sensible to replace seed oils with butter, coconut oil, and olive oil, within reason.

Soy, particularly unfermented soy, also seems to be a potential metabolism suppressant. So during recovery, it is wise to reduce soy consumption. Does that mean you cannot or should not eat small amounts of soy sauce? Probably not. For most people, that is fine. But you'll probably have an easier time recovering if you eat cheese in place of tofu and beef in place of tempeh. And use real, whole milk in place of soy milk, or any of the other seed or nut milks.

While recovery requires ensuring adequate caloric intake, it also requires listening to your body's cravings and obeying them. In conversations, I frequently have people tell me that they exercise willpower to prevent themselves from eating an extra brownie or an extra helping of pie. We've been taught that many foods are unhealthy, and as a result, we ignore or deny our body's urgings to eat. During recovery, the goal is to fear no food, obey the body's cravings, and eat as much as we desire.

Pregnancy

Pregnancy creates large caloric and nutritional demands on the mother-to-be. By most reasonable estimates, pregnant women require approximately 3,500 calories *minimum* every day during pregnancy. The key word is *minimum,* since additional calories may be required.

Human traditions going back as far as has been recorded have given great importance to natal nutrition. In fact, many cultures have traditionally placed emphasis on nutrition not only during pregnancy, but also prior to conception for both the mother *and* the father. So we can see that traditionally humans have understood the great importance of eating enough during this special time.

Unfortunately, nutritional advice to pregnant women is now being distorted to fit with the modern (unhealthy) values such as maintaining a thin appearance and eating less food to follow the recommendations of those who believe that too much food causes disease. As a result, it is extremely common now to see recommendations such as "you need only about 300 more calories per day [than you did before becoming pregnant]" (quote from Julie Redfern, RD, LDN, a registered dietician at Brigham and Women's Hospital in Boston) or "1,800 calories per day during the first trimester; 2,200 calories per day during the second trimester; 2,400 calories per day during the third trimester" (from the National Institutes of Health). And in the U.S., CBS News even reported that "Diet during pregnancy is safe and reduces risk for complications, study finds!" This irresponsible headline is based upon the reportings of a paper published in the British Medical Journal. The paper itself, however, merely states that of the interventions studied, calorie restriction reduced birth weights of babies born to women who are considered to be obese. To jump from that to "diet during pregnancy is safe" is insane, to put it mildly. The assumption being made is that reducing birth weights of babies born to "obese" women is desirable, regardless of the means by which that goal is achieved, which is a shaky premise to begin with. But the findings of such a study should *never* be generalized. No traditional cultures, including "traditional" American culture, have endorsed calorie restriction during pregnancy, and for good reason – because it's unsafe for the developing baby.

Another common and disturbing trend these days is for women to be encouraged to diet after giving birth. The Mayo Clinic suggests that it is "reasonable to lose up to 1 pound a week" immediately after giving birth, "through diet and exercise."

These recommendations are dangerous. Breastfeeding mothers require *even more calories* than pregnant women. Dieting during this time is harmful both to the mother and to the baby.

Furthermore, growing and giving birth to a baby places tremendous demands on the mother's body. Like any other stress, this (natural) stress requires additional calories and nutrients in order to recover fully. By dieting during the post-partum period, a mother risks damaging her body and metabolic health.

Pregnant and breastfeeding women, like all people, will likely do best to obey their appetites. If the appetite is blunted for some reason, then it is best to eat a minimum number of calories a day. But as long as there is an appetite, it is reasonable to eat as much as one has a desire to eat – and to eat whatever one wants to eat.

Yes, You Will Gain Weight (Get Over It)

Many people are terrified of gaining weight. We've been convinced that more weight is both unhealthy and unattractive.

But given everything that we've covered in this book, the reality may be very simple. You may have to choose between being sick and thin, or healthy and heavier.

Unfortunately, many people I communicate with would rather be sick than gain weight. I hope for your sake that you are not one of them, because it is so much nicer to be healthy and heavier than to be sick and thin. I can tell you from personal experience.

The bottom line is that most sick people I speak with are not eating enough. Not even close. Their metabolic rates are suppressed dramatically. And so when they begin to eat more food, they will gain weight. It's almost guaranteed.

Not only will you gain weight when you begin to recover, but you will eventually probably put on even more weight than you had before you started starving yourself. Remember that in the Minnesota Starvation Experiment, the men averaged an extra 10 percent in weight, and most of that was fat. So you can expect the same for you – perhaps even more depending on how long and how badly you've restricted and starved.

It gets even worse, because not only will you gain fat, you may also gain water weight. That's right, edema is not only a symptom of starvation, but also of *recovery*. It doesn't happen to everyone, but it happens to enough that it is worth mentioning. And in some cases, it is uncomfortable.

So far, this probably doesn't sound very appealing. But what I haven't mentioned yet is that along with the fat and water weight comes improved sleep, warmth returning to the body, improvements in digestion, reduction in anxiety, and general feelings of wellness. Life gets better when you eat enough, even if it means gaining some weight and experiencing swelling from water retention. These are signs of healing. So be encouraged. It gets better.

Some people gain 20 pounds. Some people gain 50 pounds. Some people gain 100 pounds. Weight gain will happen. And if you restrict, then you will prolong the suffering and likely gain even more weight in the long run. So see it through. Eat as much as you desire to eat of whatever you desire to eat. Rest a lot. Enjoy life as much as possible. Smile.

As you will likely recall, the men who participated in the Minnesota Starvation Experiment eventually returned to their pre-starvation weights and compositions. And importantly, they did so by eating unrestrictedly over long periods of time. They made no special efforts to lose weight. The weight came off without effort, apart from the effort involved in eating enough. And this points to a very important idea that is known as the set-point theory.

The set-point theory, which is validated by studies such as the Minnesota Starvation Experiment, states that your body has an "ideal" weight called a set-point. Your body will do its best to maintain the set-point. If you eat more or less within reason, your body will remain as it is. If you eat dramatically more or dramatically less, then your body will adjust metabolic rate to attempt to compensate and maintain the set-point.

Sometimes, particularly when eating too little for prolonged periods of time, the set-point will *increase*. This is counter-intuitive, but it makes sense when you understand that the body will want to maintain extra reserves for times of need, if it believes that famine is likely.

When you eat enough, your body will naturally reach its set-point. This is achieved by eating unrestrictedly to appetite. Any time there is a sense of hunger, even if you have just eaten, then obey the craving.

With a higher set-point, you will maintain a higher weight than you would with a lower set-point. Starvation (i.e. calorie restriction) will only raise the set-point even higher. If you wish to lower the set-point, then the way to do that is by supplying the body with enough calories and nutrients consistently. As we saw with the Minnesota Starvation Experiment, after enough time, the body will lower the set-point, and weight and composition will return to "normal."

So in conclusion, what is the best way to achieve health *and* weight balance? If you guessed "eat," then you guessed correctly. Although it flies in the face of conventional wisdom, eating really is the cardinal rule of health and healing. It's one rule you'll be happy to obey.

Get My Future Books FREE

If you enjoyed this book (Hey, if you made it this far it couldn't have been that bad), you'll probably enjoy many of my other books about health and wellness. And you can get all my new releases in health and wellness for free by signing up for my mailing list at www.joeylotthealth.com. It's simple, it's free, and it's totally honest and legitimate. Nothing scammy or spammy or anything else like that (i.e. I won't be trying to sell you The 7 Dirty Underground Top Secret Weird Tricks for Rock Hard Abs or Young Living Oils). It's just about free books for those who appreciate my work, because I appreciate YOU. Simple as that.

Connect with Me

I welcome your questions, comments, and feedback of any kind. Please feel free to email me at joeylott@gmail.com. I am now receiving so many emails that I cannot always reply to each one, but I do read them all, and I do my best to reply to as many as possible. For the benefit of others, I may choose to publish my response to your email on my blog or in book format. I will maintain your privacy and anonymity, should I choose to publish my response.

One Small Favor

My sincere goal in writing is to share something that may be of value to you. And I endeavor to do so while keeping the costs low for readers. The success of my books and my ability to reach other readers who may benefit from my books depends in large part on having lots of thoughtful, honest reviews written about my work. You would do me a great favor if you would please take a moment to generously write a review of this book at Amazon.com. This will only take a few minutes of your time, and you will be helping me a great deal. I sure would appreciate it.

About the Author

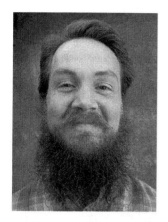

"The secret to happiness is to let go of everything - see through every assumption."

Beginning at a young age Joey Lott experienced intensifying anxiety. For several decades he lived with restrictive eating disorders, obsessions, compulsions, and an inescapable fear. By the time he was 30 years old he was physically sick, emotionally volatile, and mentally obsessed with keeping any and all unwanted thoughts and experiences at bay.

At this time Lott was living on a futon mattress in a tiny cabin in the woods. He was so sick that he could barely move. He was deeply depressed and hopeless. All this despite doing all the "right" things such as years of meditation, yoga, various "perfect" diets, clean air, and pure water.

Just when things were at their most dire, a crack appeared in the conceptual world that had formerly been mistaken for reality. By peering into this crack and underneath all the assumptions that had been unquestioned up to that moment, Lott began a great undoing. The revelation of this undoing is that reality is utterly simple, ever-present, seamless, and indivisible.

Lott's books provide a glimpse into the seamless, simple, and joyous nature of reality, offering a glimpse through the crack in conceptual worlds. Whether writing about the ultimate non-dual nature of reality, eating disorders, stress, disease, or any other subject, he offers the invitation to look at things differently, leaving behind the old, out-grown, painful limitations we have used to bind ourselves in suffering. And then, he welcomes you home to the effortless simplicity of yourself as you are.

Not sure where to begin? Pick up a copy of Lott's most popular book, *You're Trying Too Hard*, which strips away all the concepts that keep us searching for a greater, more spiritual, more peaceful life or self.

Made in the USA
Middletown, DE
22 August 2018